Childbirth without Fear:
Using the
Image Visualization Technique
To Conquer Your Fears

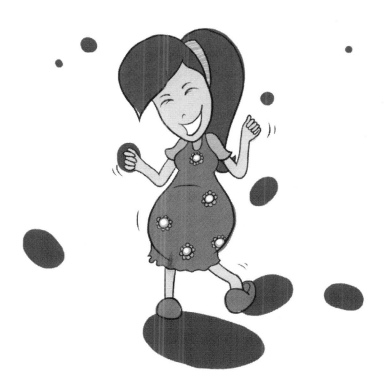

Written By: Einat L. K.

Edited By: Robert Shveytser
Image Visualization Illustrations: Neta Cohen
Book Illustrations: Leda Vaneva

i

ISBN No. 978-1630220709

First Printing, 2013

Printed in the United States of America

By purchasing this book you've taken the first step in dealing with your childbirth fears. It will assist you in having an easy and fearless birth of your child. The next step is to read the book and use the technique it introduces. I believe that the results will make you happy.

This book was written with love and care, to support you in overcoming your childbirth fears.

If you like this book, please stop by and review it at:

http://www.amazon.com/dp/B00FMWIIGE

Your success means a lot to me.

If you have a comment or question, please contact me at my email address:

contact@myPregnancyToolkit.com

My wish is for you to have a healthy pregnancy accompanied by an easy, painless birth.

Scan the following code to grab a complimentary copy of your special gift for busy women. "Your Pregnancy Relaxation Kit" is designed to deal with your fears of childbirth and help you feel calmer and more relaxed during your pregnancy.

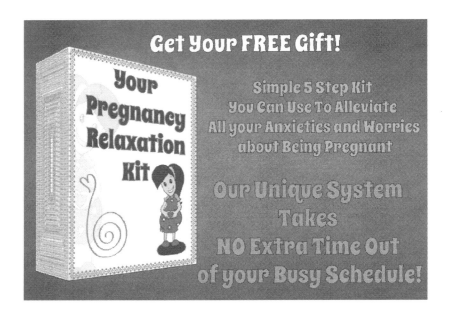

TABLE OF CONTENTS

PUBLISHER'S NOTES

Disclaimer

This publication is intended to provide the reader with helpful and informative material. It is not intended to diagnose, treat, cure, or prevent any health problem or conditions, nor is it intended to replace the advice of a physician. No medical-related action should be taken solely on the contents of this book. Always consult your physician or qualified health-care professional on any matters regarding your health and before adopting any suggestions in this book or drawing inferences from it.

The author and publisher specifically disclaim all responsibility for any liability, loss or risk, personal or otherwise, which is incurred as a consequence, directly or indirectly, from the use or application of any contents of this book.

Any and all product names referenced within this book are the trademarks of their respective owners. None of these owners have sponsored, authorized, endorsed, or approved this book.

Always read all information provided by the manufacturers' product labels before using their products. The author and publisher are not responsible for claims made by manufacturers.

Paperback Edition 2013

Manufactured in the United States of America

DEDICATION

This book is dedicated to my parents, who taught me to believe in myself and to always know that I can overcome any obstacle or any type of fear that may arise in me.

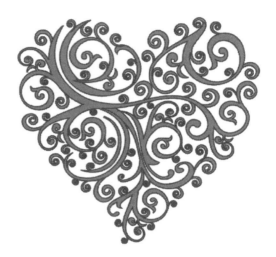

INTRODUCTION

Greetings!

I would like to begin by congratulating you on making the wise decision to deal with your fears of childbirth. Overcoming these fears takes courage, and by deciding to read this book you've demonstrated that you have it.

Childbirth is supposed to be a joyful, positive occasion, but for many women, it's unfortunately associated with pain and fear. In some cases this fear can be so intense as to have an adverse effect on the entire pregnancy. A study has shown that pregnant women who harbor a severe fear of childbirth run a greatly-increased risk of having many negative experiences during and after delivery.

Indeed, this fear can actually complicate the delivery itself. Stress and anxiety can complicate the labor process by contracting muscles and preventing the hormonal system from functioning as it should. Studies have shown that women who, during their pregnancy, suffer from fear of giving birth have an increased rate of Caesarian sections and more complications during delivery.

But don't worry: there are tools and techniques available to help you deal with your fears. If you are looking to turn your childbirth from a fearful experience into a happy one, you have come to the right place.

The only thing certain about your childbirth is that its specifics cannot be planned in advance. But you can prepare yourself for whatever lies ahead. You can learn how to cope with your fear of delivery and various other situations that may arise during the labor process.

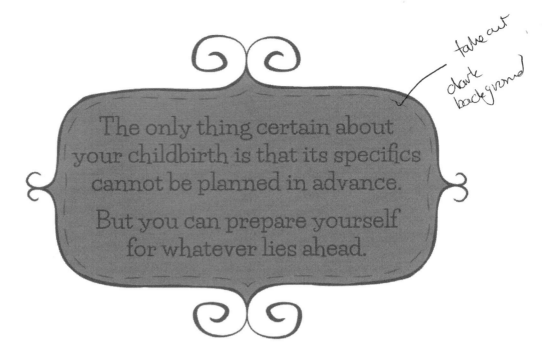

take out dark background

> The only thing certain about your childbirth is that its specifics cannot be planned in advance.
>
> But you can prepare yourself for whatever lies ahead.

Imagine for a moment that you are in the delivery room. The labor contractions have started, and now they come every few seconds. You're in pain and scared, but by remembering the technique you have learned and utilizing it, you are able to easily get over your fear and the pain of the next contraction. Your body is relaxed as you assist your baby down the birth canal. You are strong, calm and you trust in your own body to deliver your child into the world.

Your baby continues down the birth canal and is ready to emerge into the world. You are full of positive thoughts. The baby slides out easily, and the placenta follows immediately afterwards. A midwife puts your baby in your arms, and you embrace your child with love.

You did it! By believing in yourself and your body's abilities, you've managed to have a calm and peaceful delivery without any fear.

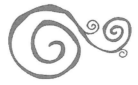

I was in your situation when I was pregnant with my oldest daughter–full of fear and concerns. How would I get through the pregnancy? Will I feel good during and after the birth of my child?

I especially feared the labor process itself. To me, the whole act of giving birth seemed threatening, and I spent a lot of time worrying about how I would be able to cope. I had heard many stories about other women's experiences, and most focused on the negative aspects of giving birth.

When you are fed such stories, your expectations tend to become negative. You begin to associate the upcoming birth of your child with fear of pain and stress. It was then that I made an important decision–one that would change everything.

I decided that I wanted the birth of my first child to be a positive experience. It would be a natural and easy birth without any fears and negative thoughts. I had plenty of time to work on myself, and I began preparing my body and (just as importantly) my mind, for the process of giving birth to a child.

We all know that childbirth is the most natural thing in the world. Even though our fears and concerns are natural as well, we can learn how to deal with them. If you decide to listen to your body instead of the nagging worries, you can make the delivery of your child an empowering and positive experience.

I worked with myself on many mental levels and used a number of different tools. One technique which I found very useful was something you may have heard of, called "image visualization." This is the technique that I'd like to share with you in this book.

Getting ready to use image visualization, I wrote down my fears and created pictures that would help me cope with and eventually minimize my concerns. Then, using the technique, I began to imagine the easy, natural birth that I wanted for my child. This eventually alleviated any fears I had of the upcoming delivery.

The time I had spent preparing myself paid off. My labor did not last long, was completely natural, and I gave birth to a lovely baby girl.

This book came about due to a wish to share these wonderful tools with women who may fear childbirth. My hope is that you too can use this technique when it comes time for the birth of your child–and that you can have an easy delivery without fear. I believe that every woman deserves a labor experience that is empowering and positive.

This book will prepare you for your childbirth by helping you deal with the **9 most common types of labor & delivery fears that women experience**. Once you have read the entire book you will be in possession of a set of tools that will help you cope with your fears of childbirth.

So go ahead and jump into the water. Read the book and get to practicing. Do your best, and you'll soon be able to see the results.

"Always do your best."

~ Miguel Ruiz, Author, The Four Agreements: A Practical Guide to Personal Freedom

"Practice creates the master."

~ Miguel Ruiz, Author, The Mastery of Love: A Practical Guide to the Art of Relationship

The visualization technique requires only a few minutes of daily practice. Since you will have upwards of nine months before it's time for you to use it, you should have plenty of time to work on your fears and prepare your mind for the upcoming childbirth.

I know this means that you'll have to take some time out for yourself each day. During that time you'll confront and overcome your fears. In the end you'll see that it was worth it–when you realize that you are prepared and ready to have a natural, easy delivery of your beloved child.

WHAT IS YOUR GREATEST CHILDBIRTH FEAR?

WHAT ARE THE NINE MOST COMMON CHILDBIRTH FEARS WOMEN EXPERIENCE?

Many women have a fear of childbirth that's greater than that of any other medical issue. Since there is a chance that complications may arise before, during, and after childbirth, it's important to deal with these fears as soon as possible.

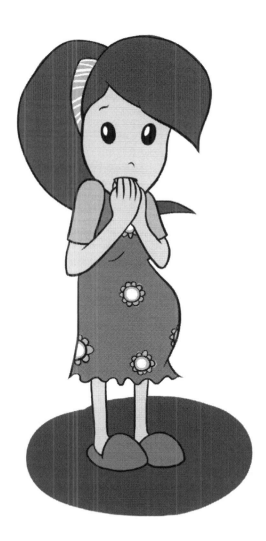

The first step in dealing with fear is to determine what it is that you actually fear. Through my research on the subject I was able to identify nine main fear categories surrounding childbirth. Please read the following list and try to identify which fear(s) you might be experiencing.

1. **Fear of pain during labor**
   Associating childbirth with pain is not uncommon, but fearing this pain can stress you out before and during your childbirth.
2. **Fear of the baby passing through the vagina**
   Many women are afraid of the tearing and bruising that may occur when a child passes through the vagina.
3. **Fear of tenseness due to pressure and stress**
   Fear of the stress itself and the tenseness that results from it is a reality for many women.
4. **Fear of the unknown**
   Childbirth is often accompanied by fear of the unknown, especially if it's the woman's first baby.
5. **Fear that the labor will not proceed the way you have planned it**
   Many women try to plan their labor in order to deal with their fears and end up worrying that their labor will not be as they planned it.
6. **Fear of episiotomy**
   Many women are afraid that doctors will have to make an emergency surgical cut of the perineum to speed up birth.
7. **Fear of complications during childbirth**
   Most women fear that some kind of complication will arise or that the doctors will perform an emergency Caesarian section.
8. **Fear of dying during childbirth**
   Some women fear that complications during labor may lead to their own death, usually because they have heard horror-stories where this has been the case.
9. **Fear for the health of the baby**
   Many worry that something unforeseen might happen to the baby during birth, or that there will be a stillbirth.

You may only be feeling one or two of these types of fear, but even one is enough to cause paralysis and stiffness during childbirth. This in turn can cause complications, sometimes requiring a Caesarian section.

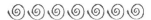

My friend Eileen was terrified of the thought of a baby passing through her vagina during her first pregnancy. She simply could not imagine being able to bring a head the size of a grapefruit out in the world. Since she did nothing to alleviate her fear, she was tense and nervous during labor. Eventually that tenseness kept the birth from progressing as it should, and she had to have an emergency C-section.

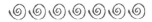

WHAT TOOLS ARE AVAILABLE FOR PREPARING YOURSELF FOR CHILDBIRTH?

There are plenty of tools available that you can use to prepare yourself for childbirth. Prenatal yoga can keep you in shape while at the same time teaching you to breathe deeply and to relax. This will help you cope with the demands of childbirth. Acupuncture can give you both physical and psychological support, and water baths or massage can help you stay calm. Positive affirmations can help influence your mind and thoughts. Reading up on the facts surrounding childbirth might also remove any superstitions or overly negative images you may have.

Every woman is different, and it's important that you find the combination of tools that works well for you. My advice is that you read up on the several various tools and select a combination with which you feel comfortable.

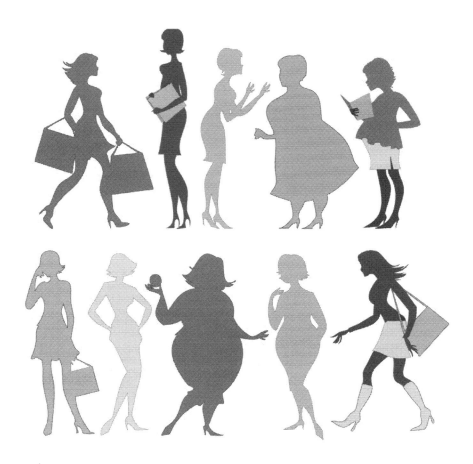

This book will introduce you to the image visualization technique, which is a practical tool that is both easy to learn and simple to implement when it's time for your delivery.

The idea behind the technique is this: You create positive mental images surrounding your labor and delivery, which will replace any negative images you might have had before. This will alleviate your stress and help you overcome your fears of childbirth.

In fact, the image visualization technique can have a positive effect not only on you but on your child as well. Dealing with your fears requires courage, and in the end you will become stronger and more confident. Your baby will sense this strength in you throughout his or her time in your womb, as well as while growing up.

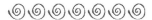

Eileen (from the example above), while pregnant with her second child, decided she wanted to work on her fears in order to have a natural and calm delivery. She practiced

the image visualization technique, where she visualized a stress-free childbirth uninfluenced by negative thoughts.

When she was in labor, her mind and body were prepared for what was to come. She could face the delivery without fear and her body was as relaxed as her mind. The birth of her child went well, without any complications.

◎ ◎ ◎ ◎ ◎ ◎ ◎

The image visualization technique is a valuable tool in your own toolkit. It will provide you with ways to work on your fear and in the end help you achieve a calm and natural childbirth.

At the end of the book I provide you with a worksheet, which will help you practice this technique. If you want to save it in on your own computer, then download it from the provided link. This worksheet will help you map your fears and impressions, and will also enable you to track how they decrease with time and practice.

Take a moment to think about which fears you are having trouble alleviating. Later on, we will work with each type of fear separately, but for now simply think about what part of childbirth frightens you and what it is that you actually fear. Are you afraid of dying? Are you afraid that there might be complications?

I believe you can overcome your fears and have an easy, simple and empowering labor.

Do you believe it too? Good, then let us get to work.

"Never take counsel of your fears"

~ Andrew Jackson (the seventh President of the United States)

Did you know?

Fear of childbirth is also called *tokophobia,* from the Greek *tokos* meaning childbirth and *phobia* meaning fear. It was first described as a condition in 2000 and may be caused by the mother's negative previous experiences, school education and postpartum depression, among other things.

HOW TO USE THIS BOOK

THE IMAGE VISUALIZATION TECHNIQUE OVERVIEW

Let's look at how the visualization technique works and how you can use it to deal with your fears of childbirth. The idea behind image visualization is that our thoughts reflect our perception of reality. By influencing our thoughts we can change our reality.

Image visualization techniques are proven to relieve pain, stress and anxiety. It is easy to use and works well for people who have trouble focusing on a specific topic or mantra. It works by harnessing the power of your imagination and replacing negative thoughts with positive mental images.

Unfortunately, the most common images and visualizations in our lives come from negative thoughts and worries. This is especially true of childbirth. Many women have heard terrifying stories about childbirth, and some have even had frightening experiences of their own. Mothers have passed on stories to their daughters and women have recounted stories to friends. These accounts tend to create a negative image of childbirth in the woman's mind that eventually gives rise to fear and concern.

A PRACTICAL STEP-BY-STEP FOR USING THIS TECHNIQUE EFFICIENTLY

The image visualization technique can be used to help you deal with these fears. By replacing the fearful mental pictures with positive thoughts, you can relieve your stress and calm your mind.

To begin with, follow these steps:

Step 1:

Take a look at the list of fears in the previous chapter. Think about each point carefully and rank how you feel about them on a scale from 1 to 5 where 1 is not so frightening and 5 is very frightening.

Step 2:

Begin with the type of fear to which you've assigned the highest number. You will start working on that fear first. If you have assigned a 5 to more than one point, simply choose any one of them.

Step 3:

Read the chapter corresponding with this fear and do the exercises every day. Give each exercise about five minutes of your time. They can be done anywhere and at any time of day.

The first few times you do it, the exercises might be difficult for you. But, if you practice them on a daily basis, you will succeed in becoming more secure and will have a stronger belief in yourself and your abilities.

Step 4:

Follow the specific instructions on how to imprint the new and positive image on your subconscious mind for each point (type of fear).

Step 5:

Every fear has a positive affirmation that will help you neutralize it. Positive affirmations can be a complementary tool for you to practice with, together with the image visualization technique. You can learn more about how to use the positive affirmation technique in my book *How to Reduce Pregnancy Stress Using the Positive Affirmations Technique*.

Step 6:

Give your mind time to absorb the new, positive images. Each fear needs approximately three weeks of practice before its neutralization will be integrated into your subconscious mind.

Step 7:

Once you no longer feel stressed or frightened and can assign a lower number to your fear, you are ready to move on to the next in line.

Step 8:

Take the time once a week to practice your earlier fear-exercises even after you have moved on to others. This will keep your newly developed positive images fresh in your mind.

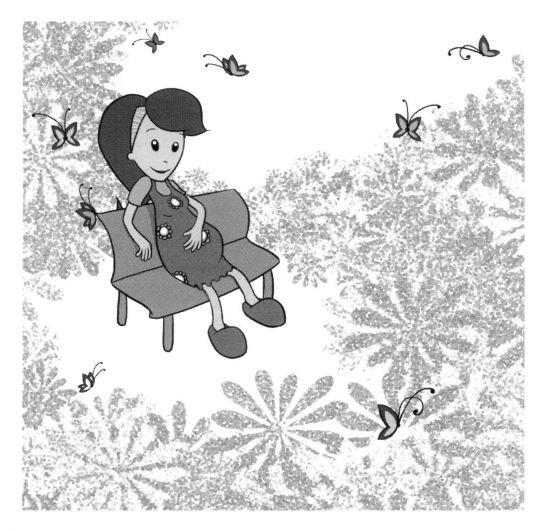

Extra recommendations to increase your success using this technique

Here are some other recommendations that will increase your success using the image visualization technique:

- **Share your positive images with your birth supporters**
  Share your new, positive images with whoever is accompanying you to the birth, whether it's your partner, mother, doula or someone else. That person may be able to reinforce your new, positive images and help you relieve stress.

- **Believe in yourself**
  Believe that you can overcome your fears and have a natural, relaxed childbirth. Tell yourself a positive affirmation every morning when you wake up and every night before you go to sleep. For example: "I *will* have a calm and relaxed birth."

- **Practice breathing**
  When you are stressed out or nervous your breathing tends to become shallow and rapid, which reduces the amount of oxygen reaching your brain and can make you light-headed and feel like you're losing control. Learning how to breathe is important in relieving stress and maximizing the amount of oxygen available to you and your child.

- **Combine this image visualization technique with additional tools**
  You can combine the image visualization technique with additional tools such as yoga and meditation. The more tools you have at your disposal, the better prepared you will be for any circumstance that may arise during the labor process. Each new tool will also help you to gain faith in yourself and your capability to have a natural, relaxed childbirth.

"You gain strength, courage and confidence by every experience in which you really stop to look fear in the face."

~ Eleanor Roosevelt (former First Lady of the United States)

Did you know?

Every time that you resist a difficult situation, you may be inadvertently giving more power to it. By acknowledging your problem, you surrender to it and can thus see the best possible solution. The universe flows in a shape similar to that of a spiral. As long as you go with the flow instead of trying to fight against it, you're following the " law of non-resistance" towards your life's purpose.

FEAR #1: HOW YOU CAN MANAGE PAIN EASILY DURING LABOR

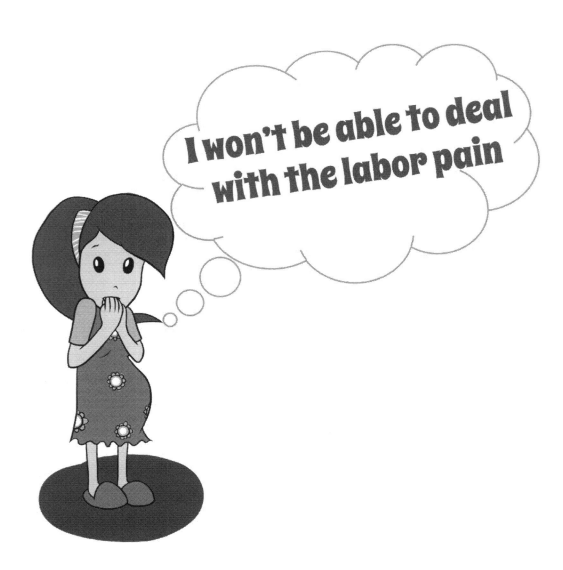

SOME INTERESTING FACTS ABOUT PAIN DURING LABOR

The birth process is always associated with various kinds of pain. Contractions of the muscles of the uterus and at the opening of the cervix are often experienced as strong cramping in the abdomen, groin and back. Some women also feel it in their sides or thighs.

In the later stages of labor, when you are ready to push your child through your vagina, the pain moves to the pelvic and vaginal area. The perineum stretches and your cervix is open. As your baby's head is pushed through your cervix you might experience a burning feeling in your perineum called the "ring of fire".

Pain during childbirth is different for every woman. Although labor is thought to be the most painful experience a woman can have, it varies among different women and even different pregnancies. Often the pain of the contractions is not what women find the hardest but the fact that these contractions keep coming with increasingly shorter intervals between each pair. It is important for you to remember that the stronger the contractions, the faster the uterus opens and the childbirth progresses more quickly.

There are many ways to help you cope with the pain of contractions and labor. Some of them are yoga, meditation, hypnosis and breathing techniques. Your body will also help you relieve much of the pain. Endorphins are chemicals produced by your body, in response to stress and pain. They are your body's natural painkillers and have a calming effect. In natural labor (without medication), studies have found that the level of endorphins increase throughout the labor process. High levels of endorphins can produce an altered state of consciousness, where you feel alert or even euphoric.

Stress, on the other hand, can cause your hormones to work against you. A hormone called oxytocin makes you feel good and triggers nurturing feelings and behavior. It stimulates powerful contractions that will in turn promote the birth of your child. Acute stress can inhibit the release of oxytocin with the result being that your contractions slow down or stop altogether.

Adrenaline is the body's response to high levels of stress, and women who feel threatened by fear or pain may produce high levels of this hormone. If the levels are too high, the birth may be temporarily stopped altogether. This pause used to help birthing women to move out of danger while giving birth but in the modern world, can lead to interventions such as emergency Caesarian sections. Staying calm despite the pain of giving birth is therefore important.

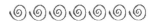

Emma, a friend of mine, felt intense pain during her contractions. For a moment she even thought her body would not be able to cope. Utilizing her knowledge of various tools to relax and stay calm, she eventually managed to give birth to a wonderful baby boy without pain medication.

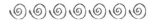

A STEP-BY-STEP PRACTICE GUIDE TO HELP YOU DEAL WITH THE FEAR OF PAIN
Practice the following to help you deal with the fear of pain.

Look at the image below:

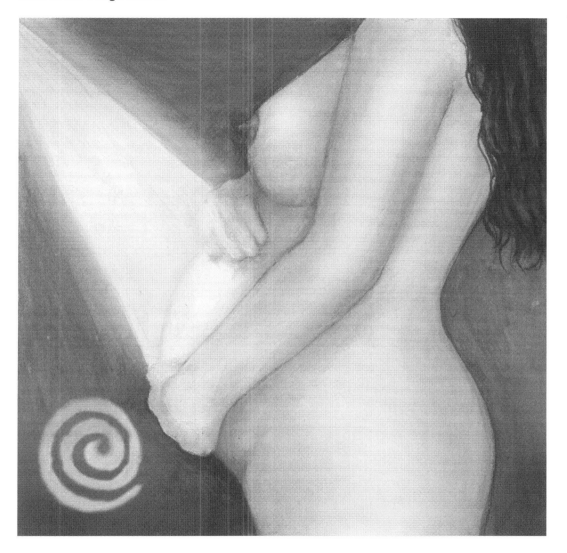

Affirmation sentence:

"I am strong and can deal with the pain by reducing it."

Perform the following steps:

1. Connect with your fear of pain. How does your body react when you feel your fear increasing? What impressions come to mind?
2. Write down these feelings and impressions on your worksheet.
3. Imagine that you're experiencing pain.
4. Now look at the provided picture for a few moments. In it you can see a beam of light that is sent to the area of pain, to reduce it.
5. Close your eyes and imagine how the beam becomes thinner and stronger, reducing the pain until it disappears completely.

You might find this exercise difficult the first few times, but if you practice it on a daily basis you will have a new and powerful tool to handle your pain. This in turn will neutralize the fear you feel related to the pains of childbirth.

Repeat step 1 once every week. Connect with your fear of pain and describe to yourself how it makes you feel. Does it still exist? How powerful is it?

Notice that, thanks to your practice, your fear of labor pain decreases. Remember that once you are in labor, you will be prepared for the pain and have a tool to overcome it.

Put the picture in a place where you can easily see it. This will keep it in your mind even when you're not practicing this technique. Have it ready when you go into labor and use it to cope with your pain.

During your pregnancy, there will be various medical checks which might increase your fear of pain, such as shots and needles, invasive tests, etc. After one month, when you have had time to practice with this image, use it during one of these tests. This will increase your confidence in yourself and in turn relieve your fear of pain.

"Pain is only what you allow it to be"

~ Cassandra Clare (author)

"The fear of suffering is worse than the suffering itself"

~ Paulo Coelho (author)

FEAR #2: HOW YOU CAN OVERCOME THE FEAR OF A CHILD PASSING THROUGH YOUR VAGINA

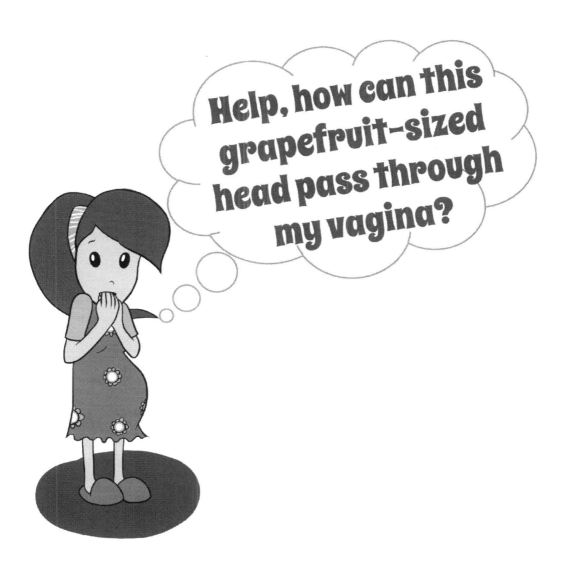

SOME INTERESTING FACTS ABOUT THE PHASE OF THE BABY PASSING THROUGH YOUR VAGINA

To enter this world, your baby must pass through your vagina. Many women fear this step of the labor process and can't picture a child passing through what seems like a very small opening. Fear and anxiety over this can cause delays in the delivery and actually make it harder for a child to pass through the vagina.

At the second stage of labor, the cervix is open to about 10 centimeters and the baby begins to move down the birth canal. This stage usually lasts for about ninety minutes. The force of the contractions puts pressure on the child's buttocks and drives the head into and through the pelvis.

This is a very intense time during the labor process. Many women have a natural urge to push as the body begins its own pushing efforts. There is a strong pressure on your rectum and it's possible to have an accidental bodily function such as the emptying of bowels or bladder.

When your baby's head becomes visible, called crowning, you will likely feel a burning, stinging sensation in your perineum. The perineal area, between the vaginal opening and the anus, begins to stretch. This burning sensation will pass when the vaginal tissue is stretched so thin that the vaginal nerves are blocked, providing you with a natural anesthetic. Your baby's head then slowly emerges through your vaginal opening.

Once your baby's head is through, the rest of the body should follow within a few contractions.

Fearing this stage of the childbirth can actually extend the time you spend in labor, according to a study. Stress hormones can weaken the power of contractions in your uterus and even stall birth. It can make your muscles tense during the crowning, causing a tear in your perineum.

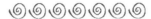

Patricia was frightened of the experience of a child moving through the birth canal and the tearing of the perineum, which can happen during childbirth. After many hours of contractions and when she was 10 centimeters dilated, the contractions stopped as she was in a panic. She was prepared by the doctors for a C-section and at the same time was helped to relax with the techniques she had learned. Before the Caesarian she was told to try pushing one more time, and this time she managed to give birth to a beautiful baby girl.

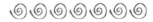

A STEP-BY-STEP PRACTICE GUIDE TO HELP YOU DEAL WITH THE FEAR OF A CHILD PASSING THROUGH YOUR VAGINA

Practicing with the following picture will help you deal with the fear of a child passing through your vagina and entering the world. Look at the image below:

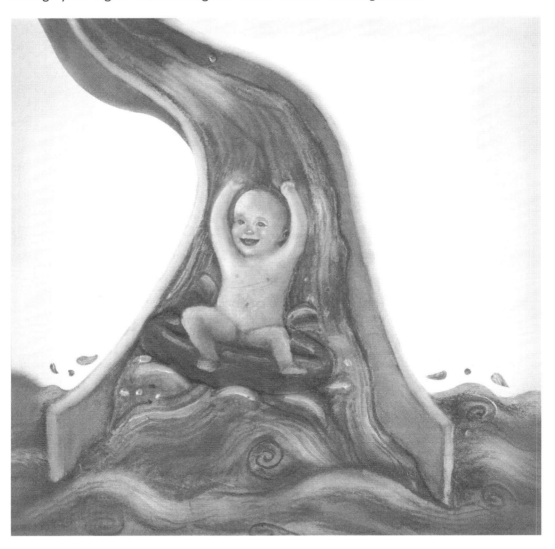

Affirmation sentence:

"My baby knows what to do and is working with me to enter this world in an easy way."

Perform the following steps:

1. Connect to your fear of delivering a child into the world. How does your body react to the fear? What impressions come to your mind?
2. Write down these feelings and impressions on your worksheet.
3. Imagine that you are at the stage where your baby is ready to enter the world.
4. Look at the picture for a few moments. In the picture you can see the water slide, with your baby riding a swim ring. Your child is enjoying it and having fun, preparing to slip out into the world easily.
5. Now, close your eyes and imagine the baby sliding through the birth canal and vagina without resistance. Imagine that the placenta is the swim ring, following the child. It all happens smoothly and in an enjoyable way.

Practice gets results! With a bit of practice you should be able to visualize your baby having a smooth and easy birth. Practice this image on a daily basis, for about 5 minutes at a time. Replace your fear with a sense of fun and joy.

Perform step 1 again once every week. Connect to your fear. Does it still exist? How strong is it? How does it feel?

Notice that your pain has decreased through practice. Think about the fact that you will come prepared when it´s time for your labor.

Put the picture somewhere you can see it, so that it will remain fresh in your mind even when you're not practicing.

"Giving birth should be your greatest achievement, not your greatest fear"

~Jane Weideman (Birth Buddies)

"Anything I´ve ever done that ultimately was worthwhile...initially scared me to death"

~ Betty Bender (speaker, Facilitator and Consultant)

FEAR #3: HOW YOU CAN EASE THE STRESS ON YOUR BODY DURING LABOR

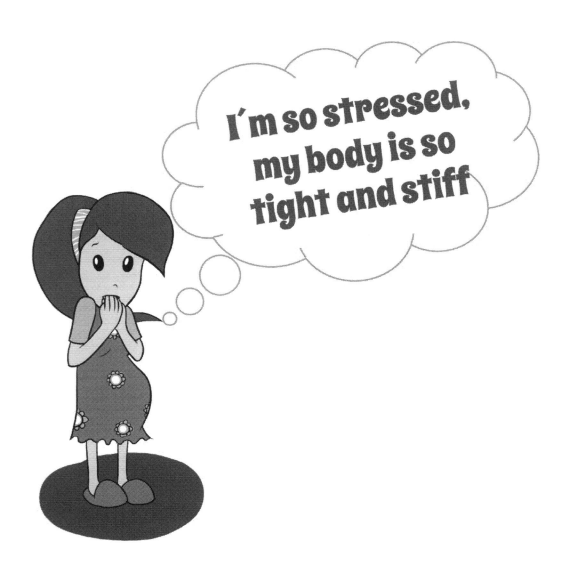

SOME INTERESTING FACTS ABOUT THE EFFECTS OF STRESS DURING LABOR

When you are stressed and anxious, you're affected by it in many different ways. Your body may become tense as your muscles contract. Your breathing becomes rapid and shallow, providing your body with less oxygen. Stress during pregnancy has been shown to affect both mother and child. This is also true for stress during the actual labor.

Many women find the hospital setting very stressful. They are usually confined to a bed and hooked up to a monitor. They may feel like they're lying on a theater stage, with an audience made up of the hospital staff. This can be a traumatic experience, and can make the woman's body tense up. Having a stiff body can increase labor pains and make the contractions harder to deal with.

During labor, you contract the muscles around your uterus to dilate the cervix and push your baby through the birth canal. If you're stressed during this process, muscles not involved in the contractions become tense as well. This means your body would be working twice as hard as necessary.

It also means that you will not be able to relax between contractions, something that plays an important part in helping the body regain strength. Your non-labor muscles require blood that otherwise would be used by the contraction muscles. The pain of childbirth then increases. This happens similarly to how the pain would be magnified if you tensed your arm as while it received an injection.

When you are stressed, your breathing becomes rapid and your body turns to the sympathetic nervous system, or the "fight or flight" response. Your breathing becomes shallow, your heart rate increases and your blood vessels constrict, raising your blood pressure.

Stress just before labor can actually stall contractions. Intense stress can cause your body to produce adrenaline, which can stop the labor process. Oxytocin then triggers powerful contractions. If you are stressed, your body might stop producing this very important hormone and lead your contractions to slow down or stop.

If you're relaxed during labor, your uterus muscles will be able to work more efficiently to give you a fast and smooth delivery. This happens because the uterus now receives the blood it needs without sharing it with tense and stiff muscles in the rest of your body. You will be able to have a less painful experience and your labor may be shorter and easier.

🌀 🌀 🌀 🌀 🌀 🌀 🌀

Eleanor was nervous about the hospital and its strange environment. She hadn´t prepared her self for having so little privacy, in front of nurses and doctors, and the area she was in was frighteningly similar to an operating room. When she came into the hospital, right away she felt her body tense up in panic. The birth was stalled due to this. The doctors diagnosed it as a failure to progress and she had a Caesarian section.

When it was time for her second child, she had learned several relaxation techniques and was able to stop her muscles from being tense. This time, she didn't require a Caesarian, and had a natural and easy birth.

🌀 🌀 🌀 🌀 🌀 🌀 🌀

THE POWER OF THE RING-SHAPED MUSCLES TO HELP YOU RELAX

There are many techniques to help you relax. For example, you can practice breathing exercises that will help you bring more oxygen to your body and enable your muscles to loosen up. You can also engage in self-hypnosis, meditation, get massages, or a combination of these techniques.

There are several ring-shaped muscles in your body, such as the uterus and the muscles around your eyes, mouth and nostrils. When all the ring-shaped muscles work together, your body will become more relaxed. Working on relaxing the upper ring muscles of your body can help you relax your uterus when the time has come for your childbirth.

Remember that the more tools to deal with stress you have in your possession, the more you can alleviate the fear of stress itself.

A STEP-BY-STEP PRACTICE GUIDE TO HELP YOU DEAL WITH STRESS DURING LABOR

Practicing with the following picture will further help you prepare yourself to cope with stress and a rigid body.

Look at the image below:

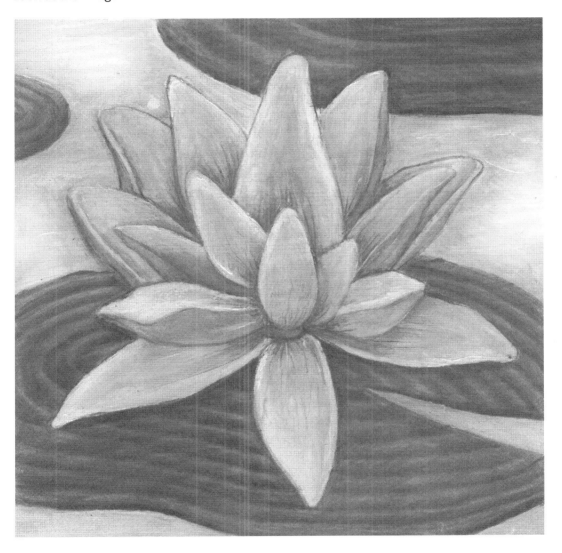

Affirmation sentence:

"I relax, I breathe, I am open."

Perform the following steps:

1. Connect with your fear of your body being constricted. Where does your body cramp? What impressions come to your mind?
2. Write down your feelings and impressions on your worksheet.
3. Imagine that your body is tense and stiff.
4. Now look at the picture for a few moments. In it you can see a lotus flower opening, and above it is the letter O.
5. Close your eyes and imagine how your uterus opens like a lotus flower. While projecting the image in your mind, say aloud the sound O. This long sound will help you relax the ring muscles of your body and gradually open the uterus. Your breathing becomes deeper and deeper.

Practice gets results! Practice this daily, and in return you will neutralize the fear you feel associated with the stress surrounding childbirth.

Repeat step 1 once every week. Connect with your fear and describe to yourself how it makes you feel. Does it still exist? How powerful is it?

Notice that, thanks to your practice, your fear of having a stressed and tense body decreases. Remember that once you are in labor, you will be prepared for stress and have a tool to overcome it.

Put the picture in a place where you can see it. This will keep it in your mind even when you're not practicing this technique. Have it ready when you go into labor.

During pregnancy many women take iron supplements. Iron can often cause constipation. You can do this exercise in situations where you are constipated to try and relieve yourself. Believe in your body. (I also taught my 3.5 year-old daughter to use this method: she loves it and it helps her very much).

"The greatest weapon against stress is our ability to choose one thought over another"

~ William James (philosopher and psychologist)

"Don´t let your mind bully your body into believing it must carry the burden of its worries"

~ Astrid Alauda (author)

FEAR #4: HOW YOU CAN EASE YOUR UNCERTAINTY SURROUNDING THE LABOR PROCESS

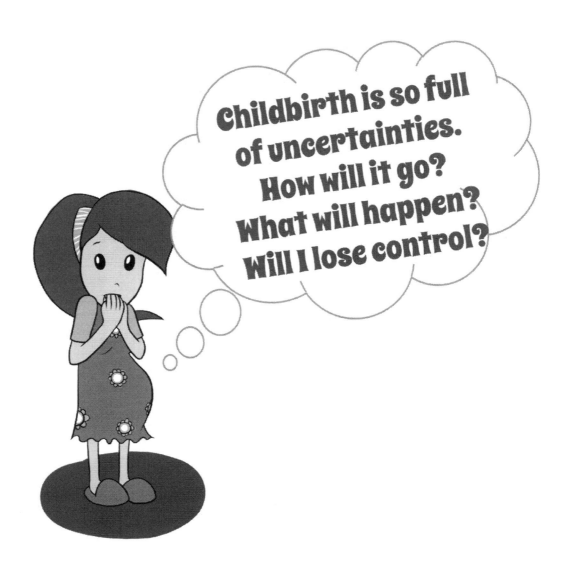

SOME INTERESTING FACTS ABOUT THE FEAR OF THE UNKNOWN

The birth of your child is often accompanied with feelings of uncertainty. It is like walking into the unknown. The feeling occurs mainly during a woman's first birth, but women who have already given birth may experience it as well.

When it is the first child, the woman usually has no idea what to expect. There are many questions arising that cannot sufficiently be answered by anyone else. How will the contractions feel? When will my water break? Will I lose control of myself during labor?

Even a woman who *has* given birth before may feel uncertain about the birth process. *Not every birth is the same*. She might have moved to a new place and needs a new doctor, or has decided to have a home birth instead of one in a hospital.

Being afraid of the unknown is a natural and common thing. It is the fear of letting go, of surrendering to a reality that you cannot control. Many are hindered in their lives by this fear. Some even experience it so strongly that they avoid doing things that might contain an uncertainty aspect, simply because they are too afraid to face what they can't control.

Fearing the unknown brings stress, which can cause an additional amount of pain to the body and even stall the birthing process. It is therefore important that you come to terms with your fear of the unknown and work on it before it is time for your childbirth.

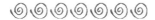

Rose was terrified of delivering her first child into the world, especially because she felt she was out of control and couldn't predict what was going to happen. In the days right before her due date she was in a state of panic, but thanks to relaxation techniques she managed to keep her body in a calm state. When it was finally time for her to deliver, she used those techniques to have a natural and smooth birth. Instead of the long birthing process she had prepared for, she delivered her baby in only half an hour after arriving at the hospital.

A STEP-BY-STEP PRACTICE GUIDE TO HELP YOU DEAL WITH YOUR FEAR OF THE UNKNOWN

Practicing with the following picture will help you deal with the sense of uncertainty.

Look at the image below:

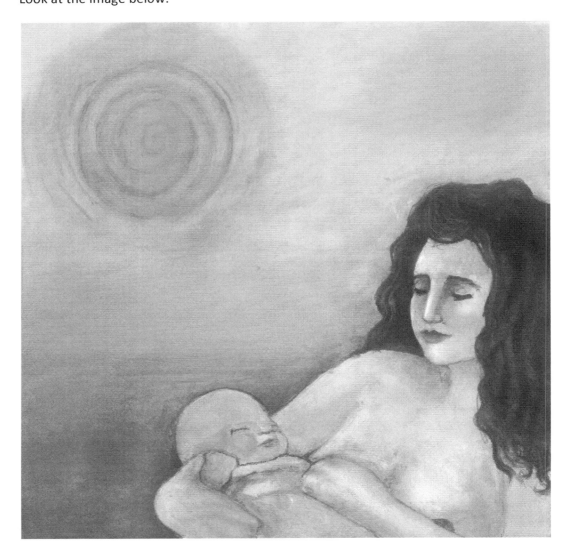

Affirmation sentence:

"I believe in my body, my body knows what to do."

Perform the following steps:

1. Connect with your fear of uncertainty and the unknown. How does your body react to the fear? What impressions come to your mind?
2. Write down your feelings and impressions on your worksheet.
3. Imagine all your fears and images that come to you because of uncertainty in the birthing process.
4. Now look at the picture for a few moments. In it you can see a woman that just gave birth, with the sun rising behind her . These two images are side by side because they both represent things that are certain and constant in our world. The sunrise is something that occurs naturally and so is your natural ability as a woman to give birth.
5. Close your eyes. Imagine the sun rising and your body giving birth to a healthy and happy baby. As the sun rises every day, your body knows how to give birth. You need to project this image over and over again in your mind, and you will start to feel more secure and certain.

Practice gets results! Practice this daily, and in return you will neutralize your fears associated with the unknown and with childbirth.

Repeat step 1 once every week. Connect with your fear and describe to yourself how it makes you feel. Does it still exist? How powerful is it?

Notice that, thanks to your practice, your fear of the unknown decreases. Remember that once you are in labor, you will be prepared for anything that might occur and have tools to overcome any obstacles.

Put the picture in a place where you can see it. This will keep it in your mind even when you´re not practicing this technique. Have it ready when you go into labor.

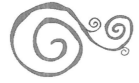

"We all have a fear of the unknown. What one does with that fear will make all the difference in the world"

~ Lillian Russell (American actress and singer)

"Unknown is what it is. Accept that it´s unknown and it´s plain sailing. Everything is unknown -- then you are ahead of the game. That´s what it is. Right?"

~ John Lennon (English musician, singer and songwriter)

FEAR #5: HOW YOU CAN STILL BE HAPPY EVEN IF THE BIRTH DOESN'T GO ACCORDING TO YOUR PLAN

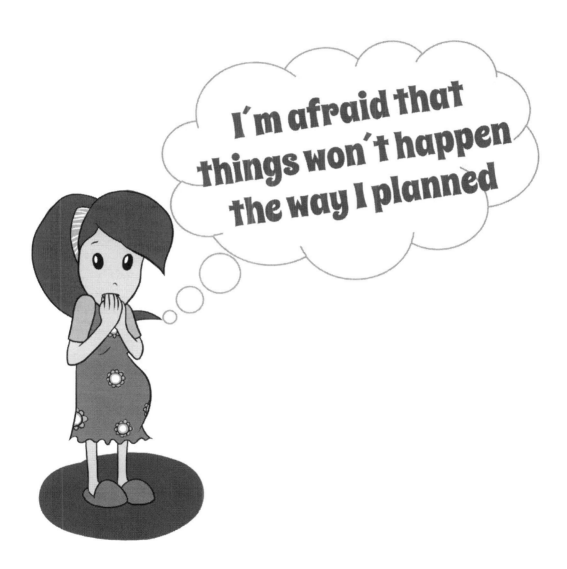

PLANNING YOUR BIRTH

If this is one of your fears surrounding childbirth, chances are you are the kind of woman who loves to plan and control things in your life. Perhaps you have read positive or successful birth stories and they made you imagine how your own childbirth would unfold. You might even have written it down in great detail. You practice different techniques and prepare yourself for labor, but the fear of things not turning out the way you want them to is killing you.

Writing down your birth plan gives you an opportunity to share with your partner and caregiver how, ideally, your childbirth would be. It gives you a place where your wishes are made clear so that your doctor and partner can act accordingly. In case you have new caregivers, your birth plan can communicate how you want your birth to be while you are in active labor.

You should talk through your birth plan with your doctor to make sure that both of you are on the same page. Go through it with your partner or the person who will be your birth partner. Make sure that they too understand how you want your birth to be.

Things you should include in your birth plan are how you will be positioned, what kind of pain relief you want and if you'd like your partner to cut the umbilical cord, among other things.

WE MAKE PLANS AND GOD LAUGHS

What you need to remember is that the childbirth will most likely be different from the way you want it to be. An infinite amount of scenarios can occur, and most births do not end up the way they were planned. Circumstances that are completely out of your control may take over: For example, there may be complications with your baby. If the birth does go the way you planned, you should consider yourself very lucky.

If the birth plan fails or is changed, you may feel anger, disappointment and guilt at the outcome. Many women whose birth was different from the plan blame themselves, saying that they should have done something different before or during labor.

The simple truth is that there was no failure and you cannot be blamed. Every birth is different. Your abilities or character as a mother have nothing to do with how your birth turned out, and they certainly do not reflect on how you will perform as a mother.

It is important that you are prepared for your birth plan to fail. Remember that any unforeseen situation can occur and you need to be ready to deal with it as it arises. Focus on the fact that your priority is to have a safe delivery and, ultimately, give birth to a healthy baby. Make the most of any situation and focus on the child you are about to hold rather than how the baby came to rest in your arms.

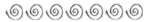

Rebecca had written in her birth plan that she did not want any pain relief, as she wanted a natural birth. She especially did not want the epidural. When she found out she was only five centimeters dilated after eight hours of labor, however, she simply couldn't take the pain any longer. She was asked if she wanted the epidural and she agreed. Once it kicked in she felt better, although she still worried she had another eight hours of labor. It only took two, however, before she gave birth to a wonderful baby boy.

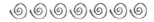

A STEP-BY-STEP TO HELP YOU BE HAPPY WITH THE LABOR OUTCOME DESPITE YOUR PLANS

Practicing the following image will help you prepare yourself to free your control over your birth plans. Look at the image below:

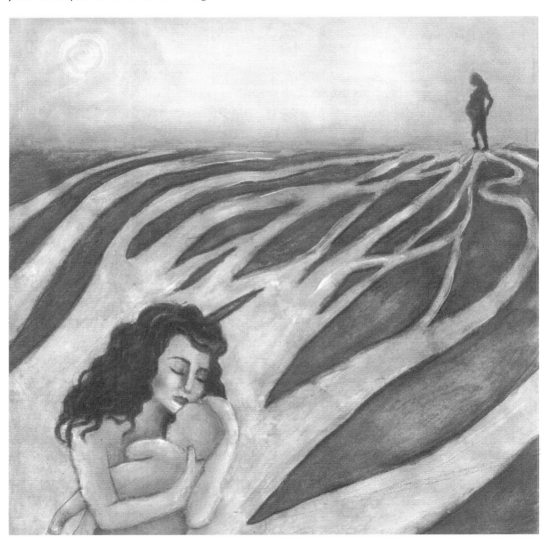

Affirmation sentence:

"I have my own special labor path, which is designed especially for me."

Perform the following steps:

1. Connect with the fear you feel when you think that your birth might not follow your plans. How does your body feel? What impressions come to your mind?
2. Write down your feelings and impressions on your worksheet.
3. Imagine that you are in the process of birth, and during this process comes a point when you are facing a different direction than you had planned.
4. Now look at the picture for a few moments. In it you can see yourself standing at a starting point of many paths. They all lead to the same end point, in which you are holding your baby in your arms.
5. Close your eyes, and imagine how you choose a path and then walk it. When faced with an obstacle, you do not stop but turn to a new path instead. At the end of the path you reach your destination, where you are happy, hugging your baby.

The first few times this exercise might be difficult for you. When you encounter an obstacle you might feel frustrated, but if you get used to it and practice on a daily basis you will succeed to eliminate your need to control your childbirth. This in turn will neutralize your fear and frustration, and you will know that you have your special path that will lead you to your baby.

Repeat step 1 once every week. Connect with your fear and describe to yourself how it makes you feel. Does it still exist? How powerful is it?

Notice that, thanks to your practice, your fear decreases. Remember that once you are in labor, you will be prepared for anything that might occur even if it is not in your plan.

Put the picture in a place where you can see it. This will keep it in your mind even when you're not practicing this technique. Have it ready when you go into labor.

"Plan may fail, life goes on"

~ Toba Beta (author)

"Nothing goes exactly as planned. Make your own destiny"

~ Tate Hallaway (author)

FEAR #6: HOW YOU CAN MINIMIZE THE RISK OF AN EPISIOTOMY AND VAGINAL TEARS

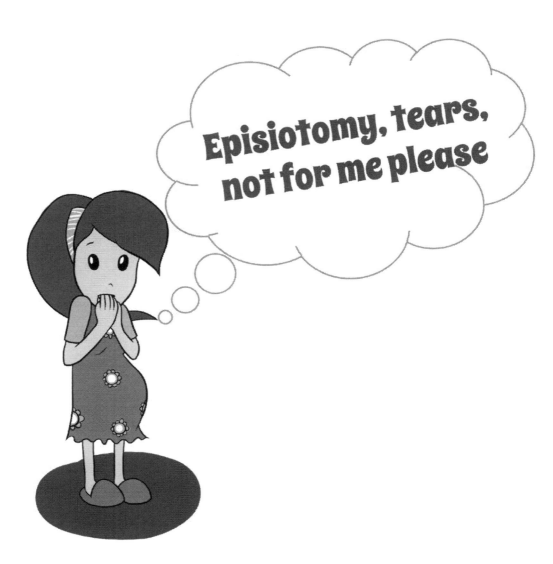

SOME INTERESTING FACTS ABOUT EPISIOTOMY AND TEARING

The vagina expands impressively during childbirth, but sometimes the expansion is not enough. When the baby´s head pushes through, it may tear the vagina.

If the tear is uncontrolled, it may happen in the wrong direction and create a jagged-cut. The most vulnerable part is the membrane separating the rectum and vagina called the perineum. Episiotomy is a controlled and straight cut that will allow the child to pass through the vagina without further tears, and it is easy to stitch afterwards.

There is bound to be some tearing when you deliver a child vaginally. Most often the tear is first- or second-degree. First-degree tearing is small and only requires a few stitches, if any. Second-degree tearing is a little deeper and reaches the muscle beneath the skin. Third- and fourth-degree tearing only happens in 4% of deliveries and is most likely nothing to worry about.

Episiotomies may be performed if your baby has fetal distress, where his or her heart rate increases or decreases before birth. This means the baby might not be getting enough oxygen and needs to be delivered quickly. If the baby´s head is already moving down the birth canal, a Caesarian section is not appropriate and an episiotomy might be used to speed up birth.

An episiotomy might also be performed if your vagina needs to be widened so that instruments can be inserted. This is most often in case of a breech birth or if you are too exhausted to push. It is also often done in order to prevent a ragged tear that will take longer to heal. Episiotomies are usually repaired within an hour after the birth of your child and you should heal within a month.

THINGS YOU CAN DO TO REDUCE THE RISK OF TEARING

There are some things you can do to reduce the risk of tearing. Remembering not to push too hard, and only pushing when told to, may help in limiting tearing. Studies have also shown that women who perform perineum massage before childbirth have less tearing than women who do not.

To perform a perineum massage on yourself, wash your hands and use a lubricant such as olive oil or cocoa butter. Place your thumbs 1 to 1/2 inches inside your vagina. Press downwards with your thumbs and sideways at the same time, gently stretching until you feel a slight burning or stinging sensation. Hold the pressure steady for about two minutes or until the area becomes a little numb.

Slowly massage back and forth over the lower half of your vagina. As you massage, pull outwards gently with your thumbs. Do this massage once a day, starting around the thirty-fourth week of your pregnancy. You can also use your partner to perform this massage.

You should also remember to note in your birth plan that you do not want an episiotomy. If it is necessary, however, remember that the most important thing in childbirth is that your baby is delivered healthy, and that the episiotomy was performed for you and your baby's sake.

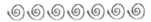

Janine was terrified of having an episiotomy and of her vagina tearing. In order to deal with her fears and stretch her vagina, she did perineum massage daily for four weeks before her due date. In the end she had to go through a vacuum extraction to get her baby boy out and only had two stitches from where the vacuum had been. This little cut healed up very quickly.

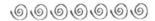

A STEP-BY-STEP TO HELP YOU DEAL WITH THE FEAR OF EPISIOTOMY AND TEARING

Practicing the following picture will help you prepare yourself and deal with your fear of tearing and the perineum not stretching enough during labor.

Look at the image below:

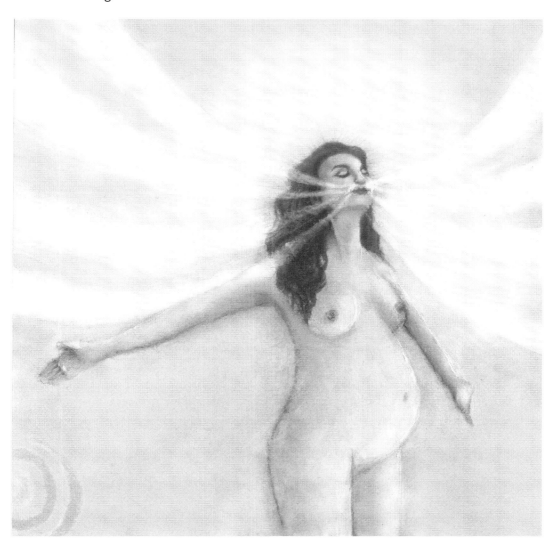

Affirmation sentence:

"I am able to release and let go."

Perform the following steps:

1. Connect with the fear you feel about the perineum not expanding enough during your childbirth. How does your body react to the fear? What impressions come to your mind?
2. Write down your feelings and impressions on your worksheet.
3. Imagine that you are in the process of birth, and that the baby is about to pass your perineum. Your perineum is ready because you did the massage to make it more flexible.
4. Now look at the picture for a few moments. In the picture you can see a woman breathing. She is calm and relaxed. Relaxation helps the perineum stretch and open.
5. Close your eyes and imagine yourself during labor. You're breathing, you're loose and relaxed. The massage did its job and made your perineum flexible. Your relaxed body helps your perineum expand and the baby is delivered without you needing to be cut.

Practice gets results! Practice this daily,and you should start to see a positive picture of your perineum stretching while you stay calm and relaxed. This in turn will neutralize your fear of needing an episiotomy.

Repeat step 1 once every week. Connect with your fear and describe to yourself how it makes you feel. Does it still exist? How powerful is it?

Notice that, thanks to your practice, your fear decreases. Remember that once you are in labor, you will be ready.

Put the picture in a place where you can see it. This will keep it in your mind even when you're not practicing this technique. Have it ready when you go into labor.

To work on your fear of episiotomy, you can also use the lotus flower image.

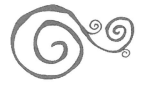

"Everyone has inside them a piece of good news. The good news is you don't know how great you can be! How much you can love! What you can accomplish! And what your potential is."

~ Anne Frank (Jewish diarist)

"In the middle of every difficulty lies opportunity."

~ Albert Einstein (theoretical physicist)

FEAR #7: HOW TO OVERCOME THE FEAR THAT SOMETHING WILL GO WRONG DURING CHILDBIRTH

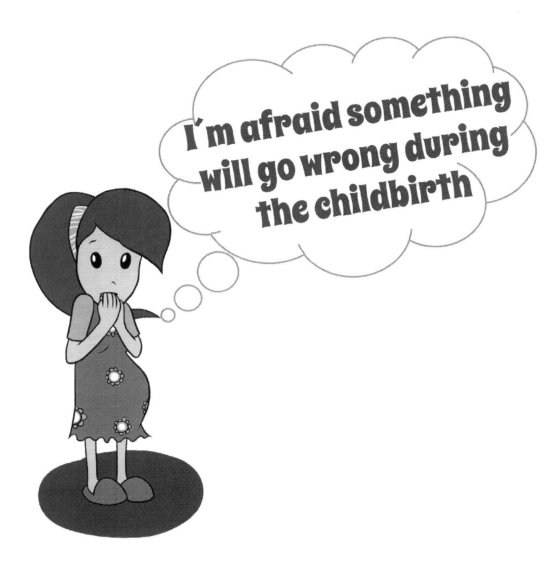

How do Fear of complications rise

You might be one of many women who are afraid that complications will occur during labor. These fears usually arise due to negative birth stories from friends, books, TV series, etc.

There are many things that can go wrong during labor, such as your baby moving into a breech position or your contractions not coming on as they should. Many of these situations will lead to a necessary Caesarian section and not put you or your child in any grave danger. Most of the situations will also become apparent before you even go into labor and be dealt with beforehand.

Surround yourself in positive feelings

A way to deal with your fear of complications is to discuss them with your doctor or midwife. A professional can explain how to avoid the most common interventions and tell you when and why it might become necessary to perform a C-section, induction, forceps or vacuum, for example.

Negative images stick to your subconscious and create a very real fear of something going wrong during childbirth. This fear creates stress and can affect both you and your child negatively. Studies have shown that fear of childbirth leads to a greater risk for Caesarian sections, dystocia and protracted labor. This means that your fear of complications can be a self-fulfilling prophecy.

You should give yourself a break from stories about complications. Stay away from women, books or TV shows that tell of worst-case scenarios and do not allow these negative images to enter your head. Choose who you listen to and try not to dwell on what-if thoughts. Remember that most interventions are done to keep you and your baby safe and that you are prepared for any complications that may arise.

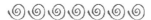

Andrea had heard frightening stories about Caesarian sections from friends and family members during her entire pregnancy. Her worst fear was to have one herself, as she worried both about the incision and the recovery afterwards. When it was time for labor, her body clenched up as she thought about the risk of complications and how frightened she was of them. The contractions nearly stopped and the doctors called for an emergency C-section. Afterwards, as she held the baby in her arms, she knew she shouldn't have worried about the Caesarian, as she realized that the most important thing was that her son was healthy.

During her second pregnancy Andrea was more confident and prepared to take the next childbirth as it came. This time her labor was smooth, and she gave a natural birth to a baby boy.

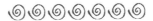

A STEP-BY-STEP PRACTICE GUIDE TO HELP YOU DEAL WITH THE FEAR OF SOMETHING GOING WRONG

Practicing the following picture will help you prepare yourself and deal with the fear that something will go wrong.

Look at the image below:

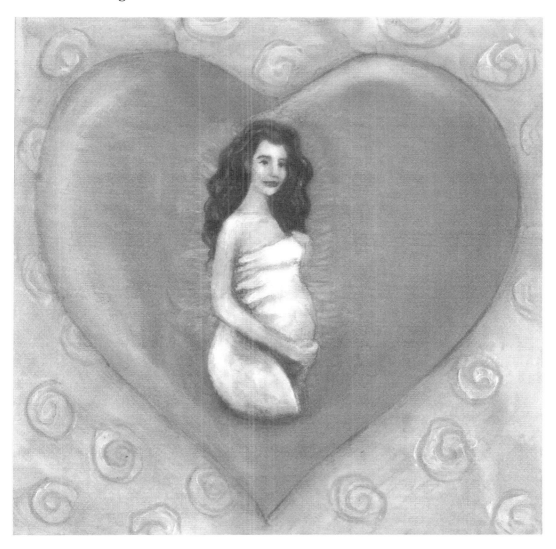

Affirmation sentence:

"My delivery is easy and healthy."

Perform the following steps:

1. Connect with the fear you feel about having complications during labor. How does your body react to the fear? What impressions come to your mind?
2. Write down your feelings and impressions on your worksheet.
3. Imagine your fear of things going wrong. What complications occur?
4. Now, look at the picture for a few moments. In the picture you can see a big heart that surrounds you with lots of warmth and love.
5. Close your eyes and imagine how the warmth- and love-radiating heart wraps around you and protects you from the complications that you've imagined. Envision yourself protected and safe.

Practice gets results! Practice this daily, and in return you will be able to eliminate the negative images and feel warm and protected.

Repeat step 1 once every week. Connect with your fear and describe to yourself how it makes you feel. Does it still exist? How powerful is it?

Notice that, thanks to your practice, your fear of complications has decreased. Think about the fact that when it´s time for your labor, you will be prepared and ready for anything.

Put the picture in a place where you can see it. This will keep it in your mind even during those times when you´re not practicing this technique. Have it ready when you go into labor.

"The best protection any woman can have...is courage."

~ Elizabeth Candy Stanton (American social activist)

"On life´s journey faith is nourishment, virtuous deeds are a shelter, wisdom is the light by day and right-mindfulness is the protection by night."

~ Buddha

FEAR #8: HOW TO OVERCOME THE FEAR OF DEATH DURING LABOR

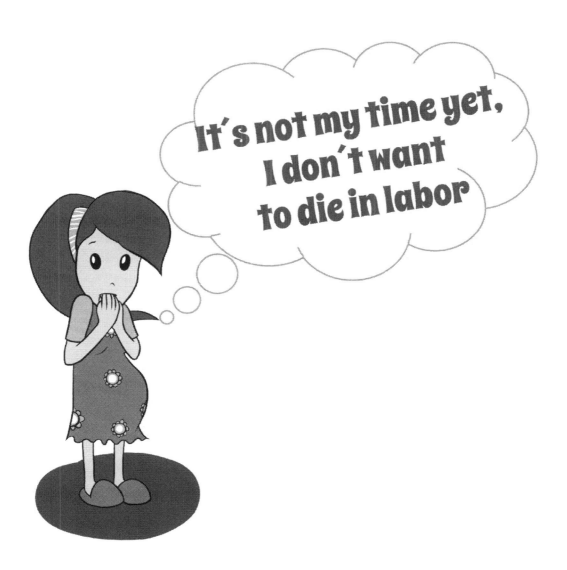

SOME INTERESTING FACTS ABOUT DEATH DURING LABOR

Fear of dying is common in people and very common among women who think their birth is going to lead to their death. Most often the fear of death is triggered by something the woman has seen or heard. A movie or TV series might have placed a negative image of childbirth and dying in her mind, and now that she is pregnant that image comes back to haunt her.

Unfortunately, death during childbirth does happen. Don't let that worry you, however, as they are still very rare in most developed countries. These are generally tied to prenatal conditions, such as pre-existing illnesses, or poor medical care.

Most deaths during childbirth are avoidable with present-day healthcare solutions. Access to prenatal care, skilled doctors or midwives during labor and support in the weeks afterwards can greatly limit the risk of dying during childbirth. Infections are limited by ensuring proper hygiene around the woman.

Births attended by a skilled health professional very rarely lead to casualties for either mother or child. Modern medicine has come a long way and professionals are often able to treat situations before they become fatal. Interventions such as Caesarian sections are done to prevent danger to mother or child.

There have been many reports recently saying that numbers of childbirth deaths are rising in the U.S. Don't let them worry you, as these numbers are still very low and likely on the decline. Recent changes in health care reform grant women who were previously without coverage better antenatal care, which should lower the number of deaths in the future even further.

If you have a fear of dying during childbirth, make sure to stay away from negative images that will empower this fear. Make sure to mention it to your doctor together with any illnesses that might affect your own health on the day of your birth.

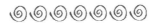

Anne was terrified of dying, feeling a sense of impending doom as her due date approached. When she was diagnosed with complete placenta previa, that feeling only intensified. She was placed on strict bed rest 30 weeks into her pregnancy and on week thirty-one went to the hospital due to hemorrhaging. To limit the risk of bleeding, she stayed in the hospital throughout the rest of her pregnancy.

Three weeks later she was able to bring her daughter home after a successful Caesarian section. She was safe despite her complete previa thanks to the competent team at her hospital.

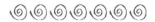

A STEP-BY-STEP PRACTICE GUIDE TO HELP YOU DEAL WITH THE FEAR OF DEATH DURING LABOR

Practicing the following picture will help you prepare yourself and deal with the fear of dying in childbirth.

View the following image:

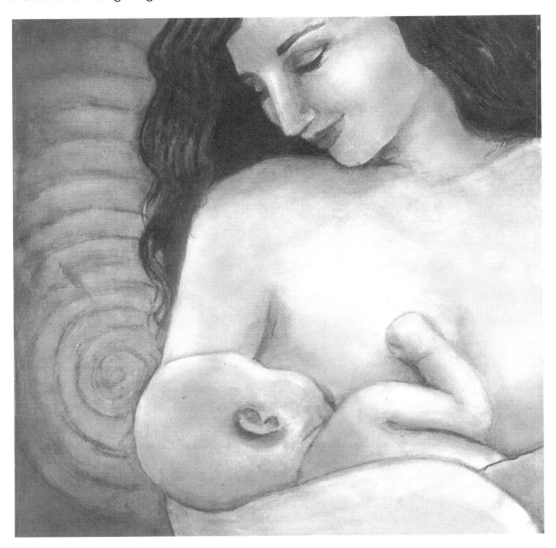

Affirmation sentence:

"Soon we will embrace our baby."

Perform the following steps:

1. Connect with the fear you feel about having complications during childbirth that will lead to your death. How does your body react to the fear? What impressions come to your mind?
2. Write down your feelings and impressions on your worksheet.
3. Imagine your fear that things go wrong. What complications occur?
4. Now look at the picture for a few moments. In the picture you can see yourself holding your baby in your arms and breastfeeding him or her.
5. Close your eyes and imagine how your baby is breastfeeding from you. You feel the warmth of his body on your skin. You are both happy and full of love. The fear of death vanishes.

Practice gets results! Practice this daily, and in return you will be able to eliminate the negative complication images and feel warm and protected.

Repeat step 1 once every week. Connect with your fear and describe to yourself how it makes you feel. Does it still exist? How powerful is it?

Notice that, thanks to your practice, your fear has decreased. Think about the fact that when it's time for your labor, you will be prepared and ready for anything.

Put the picture in a place where you can see it. This will keep it in your mind even when you're not practicing this technique. Have it ready when you go into labor.

"Don't be afraid of your fears. They are not there to scare you. They're there to let you know that something is worth it."

~ C. JoyBell C. (author)

"Every moment you get is a gift. Spend it on things that matter. Don't spend it by dwelling on unhappy things."

~ unknown

FEAR #9: HOW TO OVERCOME THE FEAR OF SOMETHING HAPPENING TO THE BABY

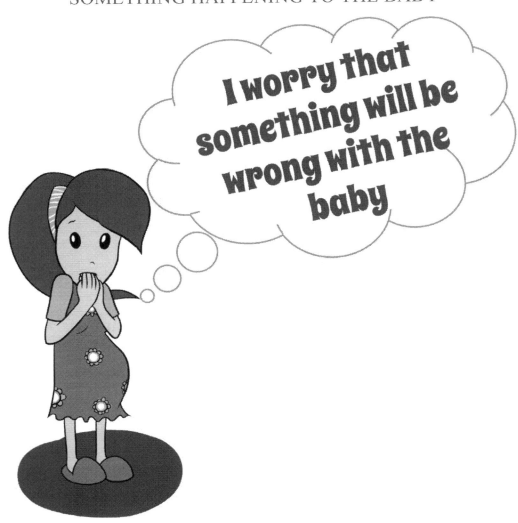

THE CHECKS THAT ARE DONE TO ENSURE YOUR CHILD IS HEALTHY

It is common to worry about your child during pregnancy. Is he developing properly? Is he in the right position for birth? Will the baby be able to pass through the birth canal?

There are many checks that are done before the birth of your child to ensure he or she is healthy. In the vast majority of cases the results of these tests come back normal. Should they be abnormal, further tests and/or treatment should be offered which may prevent any serious problems.

The doctors will check your weight and height early in the pregnancy to see if you are significantly underweight or overweight, which could affect your baby. They will also assess the growth of your child as well as blood pressure at the routine antenatal checks. At around 36 weeks they will check if your baby is lying bottom down, or breech. If that is the case, they may begin treatment to turn your baby around.

Your urine is checked for early indications of pre-eclampsia, diabetes and infections. Blood samples are taken to detect anemia (which is easily treated with iron supplements), hemoglobin disorders or infections such as HIV, hepatitis B and syphilis. The risk of passing these illnesses on to your child can be greatly reduced if treated or immunized early.

Ultrasound scans will be performed as well, and these can detect any development problems in the baby. There are also screenings offered which can tell you whether there's a risk that your child has Down syndrome.

With the increase in proper prenatal care and knowledge of nutrition, many problems that were common a few decades ago are no longer present. The chances that you will have any surprises are much smaller than before.

If you do have a genetic issue or concern, you should make sure to mention it to your doctor or midwife. Many problems can be screened for, so you can avoid any surprises.

Of course, no amount of tests or planning can guarantee that your child will be healthy. Some women will need to spend time in the hospital and others may have problems that cannot be fixed even with modern medicine. This only happens in less than 1% of all births, however, and should be rare enough for you not to worry about.

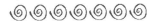

Alice was terrified when she learned that her baby was breech, lying with the bottom down. Her doctor told her that unless the baby turned before its due date, she would need a Caesarian, but Alice had always dreamed of a natural birth. Then she met an experienced midwife who told her breech births were possible. The baby never did turn around but, encouraged by the midwife and her newly found confidence, Alice nevertheless opted for a natural birth. After only three hours of labor, she gave birth to a healthy baby boy.

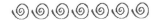

Practicing with the following picture will help you prepare yourself to deal with your baby's health concerns during childbirth. Look at the image below:

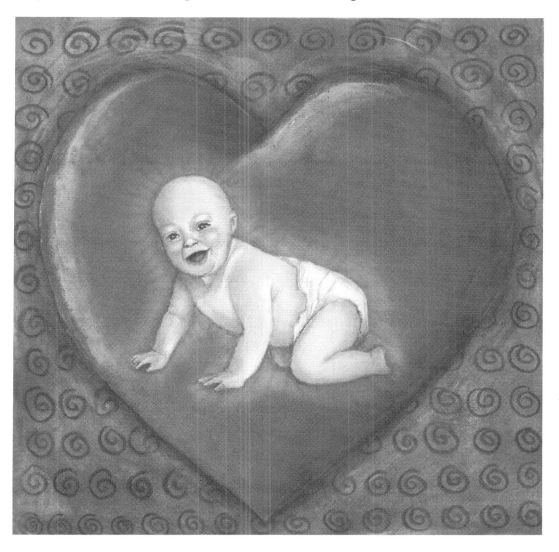

Affirmation sentence:

"My baby is strong and able to go through with the birth easily."

Perform the following steps:

1. Connect with the fear you feel about your baby's health. How does your body react to the fear? What impressions come to your mind?
2. Write down your feelings and impressions on your worksheet.
3. Imagine that you are concerned for your baby's health.
4. Now look at the picture for a few moments. In the picture you can see a heart full of light and warmth wrapping around your smiling baby who is crawling around joyfully.
5. Close your eyes and imagine the baby crawling, smiling. He is feeling great. The delivery is now behind him. He passed the birth safely and is now growing rapidly.

Practice gets results! Practice this daily, and in return you be able to eliminate your fear for your baby's health. You will see him grown and developed in your mind.

Repeat step 1 once every week. Connect with your fear and describe to yourself how it makes you feel. Does it still exist? How powerful is it?

Notice that, thanks to your practice, your fear has decreased. Think about the fact that when it's time for your labor, you will be prepared and ready for anything.

Put the picture in a place where you can see it. This will keep it in your mind even when you're not practicing this technique. Have it ready when you go into labor.

"Fears are educated into us, and can, if we wish, be educated out."

~ Karl Augustus Menninger (psychiatrist)

"Confront your fears, list them, get to know them, and only then will you be able to put them aside and move ahead."

~ Jerry Gillies (author)

HOW TO DEAL WITH A FEAR NOT SPECIFIED IN THE LIST

YOUR OWN SPECIAL FEARS

Every woman is different and experiences her own fears and worries. It might be that your worst fear surrounding childbirth is not very common and therefore not included in the list. This does not make it any less important to deal with, so in this chapter, we will look at how you can deal with your particular fear.

For this purpose, I have created the image of a pregnant woman with a spiral in her stomach.

THS SPIRAL'S POWER

The spiral shape is fundamental to all forms in nature. All natural processes move in spirals, from the galaxies out in space to sound waves here on earth. Water moves in spiral whirlpools and great hurricanes create spiral movements in the air. A spiral shape can be found on the horns of rams, in seashells and many kinds of plants.

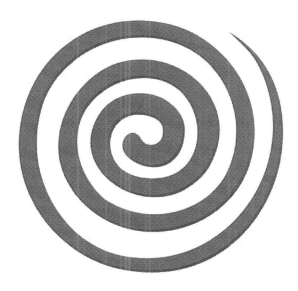

The shape of the spiral is associated with the passing of time and the cycle of birth, life and death. As a point on a spiral gradually progresses and moves further from the centre, many people see themselves progressing in a similar fashion within spiritual journeys and during times of healing.

Childbirth is profoundly linked to the shape of a spiral. Both DNA and the umbilical cord are spiral-shaped. The baby grows in spiral arrangements of organs and tissue, and during labor the child descends through the birth canal in a spiral movement. The spiral has long been the symbol of the feminine and is considered the doorway to life.

According to ancient Hindu beliefs, the spiral also depicts the flow of energy in the universe. Many use the form to meditate on or to bring energy down from the cosmos. It is a symbol of unobstructed energy flow, and using it can help you free yourself from stress and worries in your everyday life. It is a shape that puts you and the flow of your energy in tune with the earth and the cosmos.

A STEP-BY-STEP PRACTICE GUIDE TO HELP YOU DEAL WITH YOUR OWN SPECIAL CHILDBIRTH FEARS

Practicing with this picture will help you deal with a general fear you may have surrounding childbirth. It can be used to eliminate any worries you might have and help your energy flow freely through your body.

Look at the following image:

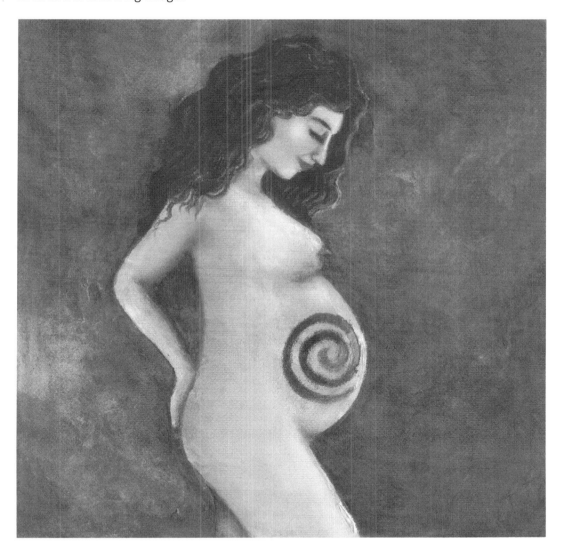

Affirmation sentence:

"I flow in my life."

65

Perform the following steps:

1. Connect with your fear. How does your body react to the fear? What impressions come to your mind?
2. Write down your feelings and impressions on your worksheet.
3. Imagine that your fear takes over you. What images do you see?
4. Now look at the picture for a few moments. In it you can see a pregnant woman, and in the center of her stomach is a spiral moving outwards.
5. Close your eyes and imagine your fears and the pictures associated with them. Imagine the spiral spinning. See how the power flow of the spiral breaks down the fears and releases you from them. Believe that you can flow beyond your fears and see how you develop as a person.

Practice gets results! Practice this daily, and in return you be able to use the principle of flow during the labor process.

Repeat step 1 once every week. Connect with your fear and describe to yourself how it makes you feel. Does it still exist? How powerful is it?

Notice that, thanks to your practice, your fear has decreased. Think about the fact that when it´s time for your labor, you will be prepared and ready for anything.

Put the picture in a place where you can see it. This will keep it in your mind even when you´re not practicing this technique. Have it ready when you go into labor.

"Life is a series of natural and spontaneous changes. Don´t resist them - that only creates sorrow. Let reality be reality. Let things flow naturally forward in whatever way they like."

~ Lao Tzu (philosopher of ancient China)

"Action and reaction, ebb and flow, trial and error, change–this is the rhythm of living. Out of our over-confidence, fear; out of our fear, clearer vision and fresh hope. And out of hope, progress."

~ Bruce Barton (author)

SUMMARY

Thank you for taking the time to read this book and to practice the *Image Visualization Technique.* I hope my book has given you another valuable tool in dealing with your childbirth fears and that you now feel like you are on the road towards a more relaxed pregnancy and an easier labor.

The book has taken you step by step through dealing with your childbirth fears.

During the process you have connected to your fears and replaced them with positive images. You shall practice these images throughout your pregnancy and use them when you need them during labor.

Practice is the important part here. Implementing the positive images and replacing them with your fears requires time and persistence. Your mind needs time to catch up on your changed images of childbirth, and you must allow these new ideas about labor sink in and take hold.

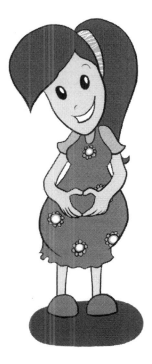

WHAT YOU HAVE LEARNED

The book dealt with the nine most common fears that women feel surrounding childbirth. Each was accompanied by an image that you can use to visualize a more relaxed birth without fear.

We first looked at how to deal with the labor pains. You were informed of how your own body will help you deliver your child naturally without stress. To help you was a picture of a beam of light, which would reduce and eventually eliminate your pain.

The fear of having a child passing through the vagina is commonly felt among women. Here you were given a picture of a baby riding a swim ring to help you visualize an easy delivery.

Next, we looked at how you could ease the stress during labor. Having a stiff and tense body can increase pain and make the labor process longer, making it crucial to be able to relax. As a visualization tool you were given a picture of a lotus flower with the letter O.

Childbirth is to many people the "unknown", and it is not uncommon among first-time mothers to have a fear of the uncertain aspects of labor. You were explained the importance of letting go. As a tool, you were given the picture of a sunrise and a woman that just gave birth, symbolizing how the sunrise is sure as nature as well as your body´s ability to give birth.

It is common for women to make birth plans, but some worry that the birth will not go the way it was planned. Letting go of control is difficult yet important since many things can occur during pregnancy. You were given the picture of a starting point leading to many paths and told to choose a new path when an obstacle occurred. This tool should help you eliminate the fear and allow you to see that you have your special path that leads to your baby.

Episiotomy is a controlled and straight cut of the vagina that allows the child to pass through without further tears. It is common to fear this procedure. However you should remember that it is done for your child´s as well as your own benefit. You were given a picture of a relaxed woman to help you relax and informed of a type of massage that could help limit the tearing, both of which should help you alleviate your fears of an episiotomy.

Many women are afraid that something will go wrong during childbirth. Although there are many things that can go wrong, worrying about this can actually increase the risk of something going wrong. You were given the picture of a big heart surrounding you with warmth and love to help calm your worries and help alleviate your fears.

Fear of dying or more specifically, dying in childbirth, is common and often triggered by a scene in a movie or book. The actual risk of dying is very low and with access to proper health care you should have nothing to worry about. To deal with this fear you were given the picture of you, holding and breastfeeding your child. You should be able to use it to remove the fearful images caused by stories and replace them with a calm picture of you together with your baby.

It is common to worry that something might be wrong with the baby. With today´s health screening processes, the chances are very slim that you will have any surprises at childbirth. You were given a picture of a heart full of light and warmth, wrapping around your healthy and smiling baby, to help ease your worries.

There are plenty of different fears, and your worst might not be specified in this list. For a fear not specified, you were given the image of a spiral and told about how this shape represents the continuous flow of energy in your body as well as in the universe. You were also provided with the picture of a pregnant woman with a spiral in the center of her stomach to replace any negative and frightening images of childbirth.

By shining a light on your fears, connecting with how they feel, and finally facing them, you should now be able to be friends with them. This is a step towards finally eliminating your fears of childbirth.

1..2..3.. ACTION! IT'S PRACTICE TIME

With the tools that you've been given throughout this book, you should be able to go to your labor prepared. You will be tranquil, peaceful, and full of confidence and faith in yourself. You will believe in your ability to give birth. You will believe that your birth will be healthy and good.

All that is left for you to do is take action. Take the worksheet and this book and start practicing. Print the images in their color version and hang them somewhere where you can see them. This will help you keep your thoughts positive and implement these new images. Labor time is fast approaching, so it´s time to get ready.

I hope that you will find your own special birth path, and I wish you a good and easy birth, without any fears.

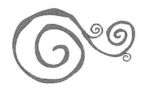

I would love to hear what you thought about this book.

Please stop by and review it at:

http://www.amazon.com/dp/B00FMWIIGE

BONUS CHAPTER - HOW TO STRENGTHEN YOUR MIND

As we have seen in this book, the image visualization technique is a valuable tool designed to influence and strengthen your mind.

Our mind is our most powerful tool when it comes to dealing with stress, anxiety and fear. Using only our mind, we can turn a negative outlook into a positive one and rid ourselves of worries. The problem is, most often we don't know how to use our minds to the fullest extent. Only when we learn to do so, can we enjoy the benefits of a strong, confident mind.

Our minds are constantly influenced by what we see, hear and read every day. Some people let every impression enter straight into their minds, and some know how to sort between what is good and what is bad for them. The difference between these people is their awareness of how things influence them.

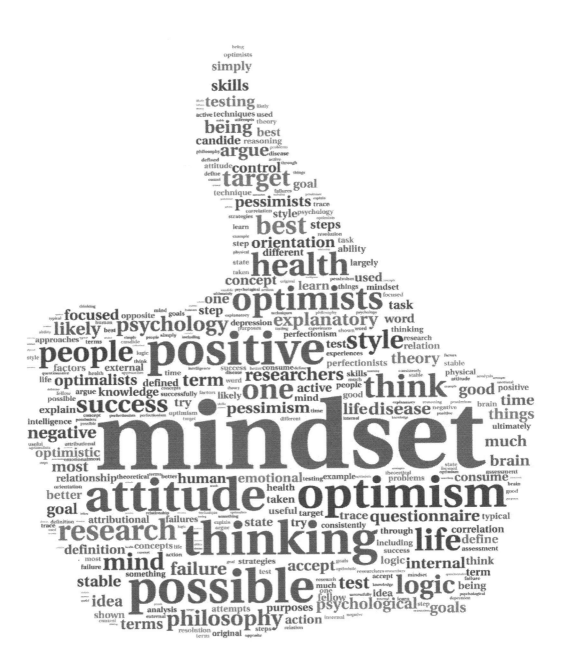

Mariah came into contact with people who told of frightening tales of pregnancy and childbirth, every day, while she was working at a hospital. Women told her what had gone wrong and how painful labor was. When Mariah became pregnant with her first

child, she found those stories difficult to ignore. The result was a stressful pregnancy because she worried every day that something would go wrong.

During labor, Mariah was terrified about the pain and became very tense. The result was that her contractions were much more painful than necessary. Only after a while did she realize that the pain wasn't as bad throughout her pregnancy as she had thought it would be. She began to relax and found that she didn't need to worry about it as much. In the end, she had a fast and uncomplicated delivery of a healthy baby boy.

⊚ ⊚ ⊚ ⊚ ⊚ ⊚ ⊚

Worry brings unnecessary stress and tension. You can rid yourself of all of this by learning more about the powerful tools that will help you strengthen your mind. Minimize bad influences and expose your mind to positive images. The more you can control your mind, the easier it will be to get what you want.

After a healthy pregnancy and a natural birth of my first child, I realized that I owed much of my success to the way I managed my mind. I decided to learn more about the mind, which is a very powerful tool, and use my newly-acquired technique on other aspects of my life.

During my quest of learning more about the mind, I encountered a great mentor, Bob Proctor. Bob is a talented speaker who teaches professional coaching seminars and his work focuses on helping people harness the power of their mind to succeed in their lives. He is also a teaching master of the Law of Attraction, which stipulates that focusing on positive thoughts can bring a positive outcome.

I had participated in a number of his seminars which were the start of a big change in my life. The most important lesson for me was **that repetition is important when talking about the mind**.

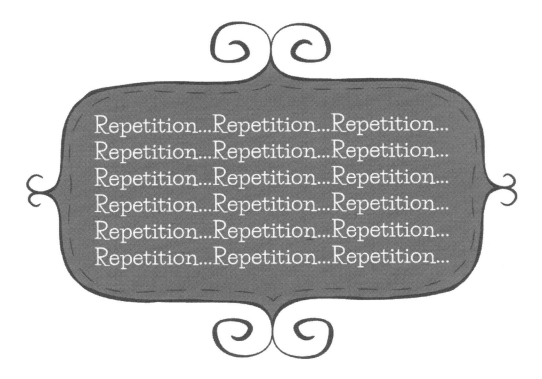

Repetition can be done in several ways:

1. Listen to audio lessons while driving in your car or doing exercises, etc. I made it a habit to listen to one lesson, every day. Usually I listened to each lesson 30 days in a row in order for it to sink into my mind and become a part of it.

An audio which I can greatly recommend is "The Strangest Secret" by Earl Nightingale. This is one of the most influential messages on audio, and it explores the question of what it takes to succeed in the ever-changing world of today.

2. Get a positive insight every day. This is a powerful tool to grow your own awareness and learn more about your mind. I like to open my day with "Insight of the Day" by Bob Proctor. By signing up for a daily insight, you will receive a short message that will give you something positive to focus on.

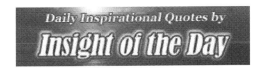

3. Participate in weekly sessions of learning new information about the mind. I signed up for Bob's streaming club. In this club I have the opportunity to meet him once a week, to learn the most efficient and valuable lessons about the mind. I've found that attending the weekly meetings is like going to a "mind gym."

⊙ ⊙ ⊙ ⊙ ⊙ ⊙ ⊙

My friend Sophia had a difficult first pregnancy and suffered from a wide variety of symptoms as well as post-partum depression. When she became pregnant with her second child, she was determined to change her mindset and have a positive experience during pregnancy and childbirth. She signed up for Bob Proctor's daily insight, attended his weekly seminars and listened to every audio book on the subject that she could find, while driving to work every day. When it was time for her childbirth she felt relaxed and at ease. The delivery went very well, without complications, and this time around, she didn't suffer from depression.

⊙ ⊙ ⊙ ⊙ ⊙ ⊙ ⊙

I hope you will find these tools helpful and that you now know where to begin in your quest to expand your mind and to find more positive influences. This will help you throughout the challenging time that is pregnancy and childbirth. Afterwards, you and your baby will be able to reap the benefits of your training, since you will have a more positive outlook and a strong mind, free from negative thoughts and unnecessary worries.

"You are today where your thoughts have brought you; you will be tomorrow where your thoughts take you."

-James Allen (author)

You can find more helpful tools in my other books:

How to Reduce Pregnancy Stress Using the Positive Affirmations Technique

SPECIAL BONUS - THE TREE OF POWER

While you were reading this book, you probably understood the importance of positive images in order to make reality the kind of birth you want. I do believe, however, that you will eventually have more tools in your kit than this. Here are some additional tools that you can include to help you be as prepared as possible for your childbirth.

Maintain a well-balanced diet

Maintaining a well-balanced diet and regular exercise are the primary things a pregnant woman should do to prepare herself for labor. Just as any runner will eat high-energy foods to prepare for a marathon, you should eat healthy food while you are pregnant, in order to prepare for labor.

Healthy fats from sources like flaxseed oil and avocados will help ensure your tissues are strong, which will make them less likely to tear. Choose whole foods whenever possible and buy food without artificial additives and antibiotics. You should also avoid soda and fries (and any deep-friend foods), as well as coffee, and make sure to drink a lot of water.

You can learn more about simple and easy tactics to prepare nourishing meals during your pregnancy in my book *Pregnancy Diet : A Practical Guide For Busy Women*

Consider doing yoga

This type of workout focuses on your mind, as well as on physical exercise and will prepare both your body and mind for what lies ahead. Yoga helps with strength, stamina and focus, which are all required during childbirth.

Yoga also teaches correct breathing. To be aware of your breathing and be able to use it against your pain is an important skill during labor, as is being able to stretch your body's limits. Studies have shown that women doing yoga during their pregnancies experience less pain and shorter labor duration than women who do not.

Do exercise

Another type of exercise that will help you during labor is water exercises such as swimming or walking in a pool. Exercising in water is ideal for pregnant women since the water supports your body, reducing the risk of stress-related injuries. It also soothes joints and muscles that are stressed by your pregnancy. Simply swimming, walking or running in water will strengthen your muscles and help you prepare for labor.

Other ways to exercise includes walking, dancing or aerobics. Make sure to take at least a 10-minute walk every day and keep a straight posture to help prevent a poorly positioned baby.

Practice Kegel exercises

Kegel exercises are also very important. Repeatedly contracting and relaxing the muscles in your pelvic floor strengthens and opens it during delivery. It will also help against incontinence and may help speed-up your recovery after childbirth.

Gather some info

Read up on any information that can help you through your delivery. Knowing what to expect will not only alleviate your fears, but teach you what you should prepare for.

Join prenatal classes

You can also go to prenatal classes. Not only do they help you focus on your pregnancy and the coming labor, but also allow you to meet other expectant mothers. Meeting other women can help you deal with your fear and stress surrounding childbirth. Doing so may provide you with new information about the labor process, teach you about medical procedures and possible interventions. You might also gather some new advice on relaxation techniques.

Prenatal classes also offer the chance to learn about and experiment with different birth positions. You will be guided in your pain relief choices as well as learn massage skills and breathing techniques.

Practice breathing techniques

Remember to practice a few breathing techniques to help you with pain and stress during labor. Studies have shown that this kind of relaxation technique is linked to a lower risk of Caesarian sections and assisted births.

Keep track of your toolkit

In order to help you keep track of your many different tools, I have included a copy of the "Tree of power" as a special bonus to this book. You can print it and write down all the positive assets and tools that you have for the upcoming labor. Hang it in front of you and look at it often, especially if you have any doubts about the upcoming labor. You should also put a copy of it in your birth bag in case you need it to give you strength at some point in the future.

Attached is an example of my pregnancy tree of power:

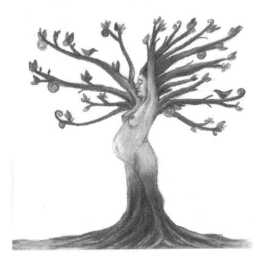

My Pregnancy Tree of Power

My positive assets and tools that I have for my upcoming childbirth

1. Weekly exercise of prenatal yoga

2. Practice breathing techniques

3. Cope with my childbirth fears with the Image visualization technique & the Positive affirmations technique

4. Perform a perineum massage by my partner

5. Maintaining a well-balanced diet

6. Acupuncture treatments once a month

Scan the code below to download your free copy of the your tree of power .

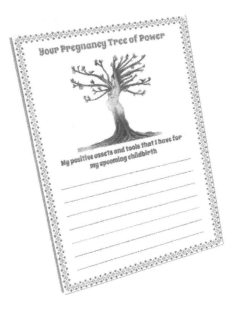

I hope you have enjoyed this book and now feel that you have an additional tool in your kit when the time comes for your labor. I wish you a relaxed, natural and calm birth.

A WORKSHEET WHICH WILL HELP YOU PRACTICE THE TECHNIQUE

Here are the examples of the worksheet that you can use to help you practice the technique.

Your Practice Worksheet

Please rank on a scale from 1 to 5 how you feel about each fear listed below, where 1 is not so frightening and 5 is very frightening.

		Fear type	How do you feel about the fear? 1- not so frightening 5 - very frightening	Start date of working on the fear	Did I complete the main exercise of the fear *Each fear needs approximately three weeks of practice before its neutralization will be integrated into your subconscious mind
1		Fear of pain during labor			
2		Fear of the baby passing through the vagina			
3		Fear of tenseness due to pressure and stress			
4		Fear of the unknown			
5		Fear that the labor will not proceed the way			

Fear: _____

Exercise Day #	Exercise date	How does your body react to the fear? Where do you feel it in your body? Write down your feelings and impressions	Does the fear still exist?	How powerful is the fear? 0 - vanished 1- not so frightening 5 - very frightening
1.				
2.				
3.				
4.				
5.				
6.				

You can use these examples to create your own worksheet, or scan the code below to download these templates.

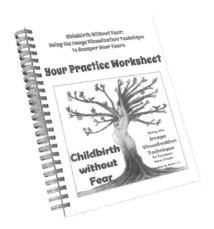

Have a fun practice!

ABOUT THE AUTHOR

Einat is a mother to a lovely girl.
She has been studying for the last 15 years the powerful ways to use your mind & subconscious and live a quiet, peaceful and better life.
She tries to live according to the methods she's learned in all areas of her life.

Einat believes in the principles of flow , liberation and positive thinking.
That's why she loves the shape of the spiral.
She implements these principles in her daily life.
She's on an endless journey of her personal development and tries to do the best she can.

When she became pregnant with her first daughter, she implemented the tools she learned about herself in order to have an easy, pleasant and empowering pregnancy.

Einat had many concerns about the birth process but with the tools and techniques which she applied to herself she was able to overcome these concerns and gave a natural childbirth to a healthy daughter.

Einat is the co-founder of a new pregnancy web site www.myPregnancyToolkit.com that brings a set of practical tools for pregnant women that focuses on the pregnancy issues from the mind's perspective.

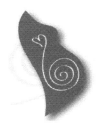
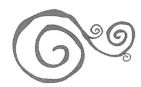

MORE BOOKS AND PRODUCTS BY THE AUTHOR

Childbirth without Fear - Guided Meditations to help you Conquer Your Fears

The *audio guided meditations* are part of a set of helpful tools that can help you eliminate your upcoming childbirth fears. These meditations can serve as a stand alone tool and also as a complement to the book *Childbirth without Fear: Using the Image Visualization Technique to Conquer Your Fears*. They are easy to practice and can be used any time and anywhere.

The audio guided meditations are available on Amazon.

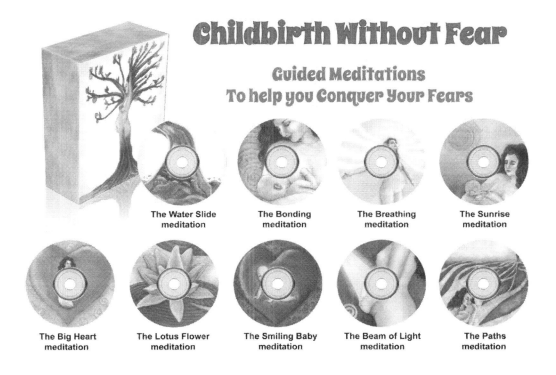

Pregnancy Diet: A Practical Guide for Busy Women

In this book you will learn about simple and easy tactics for preparing nourishing meals during your pregnancy, so that you and your baby can enjoy a healthy pregnancy.

The book is available on Amazon.

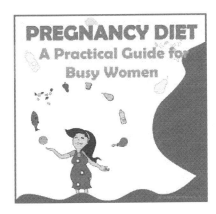

How to Reduce Pregnancy Stress Using the Positive Affirmations Technique

In this book you will learn about the positive affirmations technique and how it can give you and your baby a happy, healthy glow inside and out and reduce the stress you might feel during your pregnancy.

The book is available on Amazon.

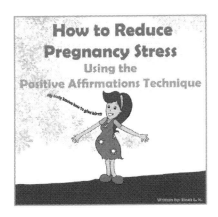

25444532R00052